Provided as an educational service by

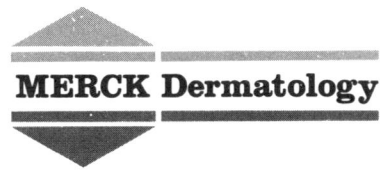

Self-Assessment in Dermatology

K. M. MOKBEL
MBBS (London)
The London Hospital
Whitechapel

WRIGHTSON BIOMEDICAL PUBLISHING LTD
Petersfield

Copyright © 1990 by Wrightson Biomedical Publishing Ltd

All rights reserved

No part of this book may be reproduced by any means, or transmitted, or translated into machine language without the written permission of the publisher.

British Library Cataloguing in Publication Data
Mokbel, K. M. (Kefah M.)
   Self-assessment in dermatology
   1. Medicine. Dermatology
   I. Title
   616.5

ISBN 1 871816 09 2

Typeset by AdServices, Chichester, West Sussex
Printed in Great Britain by Biddles Ltd, Guildford

Foreword

Dermatology lends itself well to examination of factual information by multiple choice questioning. In an essay assessment, the examiner has to search the paragraphs for relevant facts and opinions and the examinee can take cover behind the smokescreen of language. No such cover is provided by multiple choice questioning which not only allows electronic marking but also offers the keen student a fine stone on which to sharpen his knife of knowledge.

Kefah Mokbel's compendium of 220 MCQs is a remarkable collection, all the more so for having been assembled and designed by a senior medical student and not an experienced dermatologist. He has produced a collection well suited to medical students, junior (and indeed senior) hospital doctors and general practitioners interested in increasing and focusing their dermatological knowledge.

Dermatological diagnosis requires the development of visual memory skills for the recognition of many characteristic disease reaction patterns but, without a firm basis of factual knowledge, visual skills have little value.

Kefah Mokbel has provided us with a valuable collection of MCQs which contributes significantly to the corpus of teaching material available to those interested in clinical dermatology. It deserves to be widely used.

HARVEY BAKER MD FRCP
Consultant Dermatologist
Head, Department of Dermatology
The London Hospital

Preface

The MCQ format is the mainstay of self-assessment of factual knowledge. It has been extensively used in undergraduate and postgraduate examinations because of its objectivity and accuracy. The MCQ format can expose our areas of ignorance or give us confidence by demonstrating areas of relative strength.

The aim of this book, in addition to self-assessment, is to provide an enjoyable method of revising and learning dermatology, and to act as a basis for further study and reading.

I hope that this book will be found helpful by medical students, GPs and junior doctors.

How to use this book

The book contains 220 questions with answers and explanations. The standard notation is used: **T** (true) and **F** (false). An initial statement is followed by five possible completions each of which must be correctly identified as **T** or **F**. In the exam a correct answer gains one mark, an incorrect answer is penalized by the deduction of one mark, and an unanswered completion gains nothing. Remember that choosing not to answer a question, when you do not know the answer is in itself a choice.

Some MCQ terms translated

'Usually' = more than 50%
'Rarely' = less than 5%
'Never' = 0%   these terms are hardly ever used
'Always' = 100%   in good MCQs
'Characteristic' = refers to a feature which if absent would cause the diagnosis to be in doubt
'Pathognomonic' = refers to a feature which is found in that disorder and no other
'Associated' = more frequent than by chance
'Commonly' = difficult to interpret; probably >5–30%
'The majority' = >60%

Acknowledgements

I wish to thank Dr Harvey Baker for his thoughtful Foreword and encouragement. I am also indebted to Dr Julia Newton (Consultant Dermatologist), Dr F. Tatnall, Dr C. Proby, Dr M. Glover and Dr J. Salisbury for reading through the manuscript and offering many helpful suggestions.

The acknowledgements would be incomplete without mentioning Mr J. McIlree (E. Merck) and Ms Judy Wrightson whose efforts made the whole publication possible.

I wish to thank, last but not least, my parents for their remarkable support.

K.M. MOKBEL
May 1990, London

The Questions

1. **The following dermatoses typically affect the trunk**
    (a) pityriasis rosea
    (b) pityriasis versicolor
    (c) keratoderma blennorrhagicum
    (d) guttate psoriasis
    (e) acute pompholyx

2. **Dermatitis herpetiformis**
    (a) is associated with gastrointestinal symptoms in about 60% of cases
    (b) is an itchy skin disorder
    (c) can be improved by gluten-free diet
    (d) lesions can affect the scalp
    (e) responds to steroids

3. **Pyoderma gangrenosum is associated with**
    (a) ulcerative colitis
    (b) Crohn's disease
    (c) rheumatoid arthritis
    (d) Gardner's syndrome
    (e) IgA-paraproteinaemia

4. **Leg ulcers may be found in**
    (a) sickle cell anaemia
    (b) tabes dorsalis
    (c) pityriasis amiantacea
    (d) polyarteritis nodosa
    (e) ulcerative colitis

5. **Seborrhoeic warts**
    (a) arise from the sebaceous glands
    (b) are common in people over the age of 50 years
    (c) are found most commonly on the trunk and temples
    (d) are pre-malignant
    (e) may be mistaken for malignant melanoma

6. **The following statements are correct**
    (a) erythrasma responds to oral erythromycin
    (b) trichomycosis axillaris responds to clotrimazole
    (c) erysipelas is best treated by i.m. penicillin
    (d) sycosis barbae responds to antibiotics
    (e) a carbuncle is best treated with topical antibiotics

7. **Pityriasis rosea**
    (a) commonly involves the face and the scalp
    (b) is usually a self-limiting condition
    (c) is exacerbated by UVR
    (d) is usually associated with a positive Wasserman reaction (WR) test
    (e) is characterized by shagreen patch

8. **The following conditions may result in scarring alopecia**
    (a) discoid lupus erythematosus
    (b) sarcoidosis
    (c) radiotherapy
    (d) herpes zoster infection of the scalp
    (e) lichen planus

9. **Eczema**
    (a) discoid eczema commonly affects the flexor surfaces of the limbs
    (b) asteatotic eczema is associated with thyrotoxicosis
    (c) seborrhoeic eczema is related to an abnormality in the seborrhoeic glands
    (d) there is an association with Wiskott–Aldrich syndrome
    (e) napkin eczema should be treated with potent steroids applied locally

10. **Cutaneous manifestations of diabetes mellitus include**
    (a) granuloma annulare
    (b) erythema ab igne
    (c) boils
    (d) xanthomata on the buttocks
    (e) erythema marginatum

11. **The following may be cutaneous markers of malignancy**
    (a) acquired ichthyosis
    (b) superficial thrombophlebitis
    (c) recurrent facial flushing
    (d) necrolytic migratory erythema
    (e) erythema gyratum repens

12. **The following associations are correct**
    (a) ichthyosis vulgaris — X-linked inheritance
    (b) tuberous sclerosis — rhabdomyosarcoma
    (c) erythroderma — collapsing pulse
    (d) acute intermittent porphyria — photosensitivity
    (e) alopecia areata — vitiligo

13. **The following dermatoses typically affect the extensor surfaces of the limbs**
    (a) atopic eczema
    (b) psoriasis
    (c) pityriasis rosea
    (d) discoid eczema
    (e) dermatitis herpetiformis

14. **Cutaneous manifestations of rheumatoid disease include**
    (a) purpura
    (b) pyoderma gangrenosum
    (c) palmar erythema
    (d) thickened skin due to excessive abnormal collagen
    (e) pressure sores

15. **Etretinate**
    (a) is an aromatic retinoid
    (b) is free from side-effects
    (c) can be safely given to pregnant women
    (d) produces a dramatic response in ichthyosiform erythroderma
    (e) is effective in Darier's disease

16. **Köebner's phenomenon is seen in**
    (a) lichen planus
    (b) viral warts
    (c) psoriasis
    (d) molluscum contagiosum
    (e) Queyrat's erythroplasia

17. **Ichthyosis is associated with the following**
    (a) leprosy
    (b) rosacea
    (c) Hodgkin's lymphoma
    (d) seborrhoeic warts
    (e) panhypopituitarism

18. **The following are blistering diseases**
    (a) dermatitis herpetiformis
    (b) porphyria cutanea tarda
    (c) acute intermittent porphyria
    (d) pemphigus vulgaris
    (e) erythema multiforme

19. **Dermatitis artefacta lesions**
    (a) are self-inflicted
    (b) can be simulated by porphyria cutanea tarda
    (c) can be inflicted by the patient to gain admission to hospital
    (d) are more common in men
    (e) respond to local steroid application twice daily

20. **Chronic discoid lupus**
    (a) diagnosis is usually confirmed by measuring IgG levels in serum
    (b) inflammation as well as scarring respond well to steroids
    (c) hyperkeratosis and follicular plugging are characteristic
    (d) over 50% of cases progress to systemic lupus erythematosus
    (e) is a cause of scarring alopecia

21. **Erythrasma**
    (a) is caused by *Streptococcus pyogenes*
    (b) is often associated with diabetes mellitus
    (c) produces a coral pink fluorescence in the affected areas with Wood's light
    (d) responds to steroids
    (e) typically causes discoloration affecting axillae and groins

22. **Photodermatitis may be produced by**
    (a) thiazides
    (b) tetracycline
    (c) nicotine acid deficiency
    (d) sulphonamides
    (e) chlorpromazine

23. **Xanthomata are recognized features of**
    (a) the nephrotic syndrome
    (b) type IIa hyperlipoproteinaemia
    (c) hypothyroidism
    (d) diabetes mellitus
    (e) cutaneous porphyria tarda

24. **Livedo reticularis may be found in**
    (a) tuberculosis
    (b) thrombocytopaenia
    (c) polyarteritis nodosa
    (d) hypoparathyroidism
    (e) rheumatoid arthritis

25. **Parasitophobia**
    (a) responds to metronidazole
    (b) usually presents as a complaint of itching and crawling sensation of skin
    (c) responds dramatically to pimozide
    (d) is a delusion of infestation
    (e) usually has a good prognosis

26. **Griseofulvin**
    (a) should be taken before meals
    (b) is bacteriostatic as well as fungistatic
    (c) is effective against yeasts
    (d) is effective topically
    (e) is contra-indicated in pregnancy

27. **Telangiectasia is found as a result of**
    (a) steroid ointment therapy
    (b) rosacea
    (c) venous hypertension
    (d) scurvy
    (e) Osler–Weber–Rendu syndrome

28. **Herpes zoster**
    (a) mainly affects children
    (b) causes severe pain which may precede the appearance of vesicular rash by 48 hours
    (c) can be complicated by keratitis
    (d) never involves the meninges
    (e) only involves the sensory roots

29. **Common warts**
    (a) are caused by an RNA virus
    (b) usually affect the trunk
    (c) resistant cases can be treated by intralesional injection of bleomycin solution
    (d) usually resolve spontaneously within two years
    (e) can be treated by freezing with liquid nitrogen

30. Recognized causes of Raynaud's phenomenon include
    (a) systemic sclerosis
    (b) Buerger's disease
    (c) vinyl chloride poisoning
    (d) syringomyelia
    (e) nifedipine

31. The following favours a good prognosis in melanoma
    (a) male sex
    (b) a low Breslow thickness
    (c) amelanosis
    (d) involvement of trunk
    (e) regional lymphadenopathy

32. The following conditions may give rise to koilonychia
    (a) nail–patella syndrome
    (b) diabetes mellitus
    (c) iron deficiency anaemia
    (d) alopecia areata
    (e) excessive ingestion of sulphur-containing amino acids

33. Albinos
    (a) may have nystagmus
    (b) lack the enzyme phenylalanine hydroxylase
    (c) have a high incidence of squamous cell carcinoma
    (d) have pale blond hair
    (e) usually transmit the disorder in an autosomal dominant fashion

34. Immunofluorescence testing shows a linear band of fluorescence in a piece of skin from
    (a) pemphigus vulgaris blisters
    (b) bullous pemphigoid blisters
    (c) linear IgA disease
    (d) areas of clinically normal skin in chronic discoid lupus erythematosus
    (e) areas of clinically normal skin in systemic lupus erythematosus

35. The following associations are correct
    (a) Stevens–Johnson syndrome — sulphonamides
    (b) erythema nodosum — contraceptive pill
    (c) photosensitivity — tetracyclines
    (d) alopecia — warfarin
    (e) exfoliative dermatitis — gold

36. **Localized patchy hair loss is commonly caused by**
    (a) follicular lichen planus
    (b) telogen effluvium
    (c) fungal infections
    (d) iron deficiency
    (e) alopecia areata

37. **Cutaneous pruritus is found in**
    (a) hyperthyroidism
    (b) hypothyroidism
    (c) drug abuse
    (d) haemochromatosis
    (e) lymphoma

38. **PUVA has the following side-effects**
    (a) an increased incidence of squamous cell carcinoma
    (b) cataracts
    (c) pruritus
    (d) mycosis fungoides
    (e) liver and marrow toxicity

39. **The following skin lesions are characteristic of tuberous sclerosis**
    (a) shagreen patch
    (b) paraungual fibromas
    (c) herald patch
    (d) adenoma sebaceum
    (e) elliptical white macules on the trunk

40. **The following are different patterns of seborrhoeic eczema**
    (a) intertrigo
    (b) dandruff
    (c) pityriasis rosea
    (d) tinea corporis
    (e) small red patches with scaling on the trunk

41. **Cutaneous manifestations of sarcoidosis include**
    (a) lupus pernio
    (b) adenoma sebecum
    (c) necrobiosis lipoidica
    (d) non-caseating granulomas in scars
    (e) erythema nodosum

42. **The following are recognized causes of hirsutism**
    (a) polycystic ovaries
    (b) Addison's disease
    (c) Turner's syndrome
    (d) lichen planus
    (e) congenital adrenal hyperplasia

43. **Erythema nodosum**
    (a) affects men more commonly
    (b) is effectively treated with steroids
    (c) is characterized by painful non-ulcerating nodules on the shins
    (d) may be associated with a positive Mantoux test
    (e) is an example of polymorph vasculitis

44. **Port wine stain**
    (a) is usually found on the face
    (b) is occasionally associated with neurological defects
    (c) tends to improve with age
    (d) is best treated surgically
    (e) can be treated by laser technology

45. **The differential diagnoses of rosacea include**
    (a) acne vulgaris
    (b) lupus erythematosus
    (c) photosensitivity
    (d) pityriasis rosea
    (e) peri-oral dermatitis

46. **Cutaneous manifestations of hypothyroidism include**
    (a) hyperhidrosis
    (b) diffuse hair loss
    (c) pruritus
    (d) fine hair
    (e) pyoderma gangrenosum

47. **The following are associated with gastrointestinal disease**
    (a) acrodermatitis enteropathica
    (b) pyoderma gangrenosum
    (c) Gardner's syndrome
    (d) erythema nodosum
    (e) dermatitis herpetiformis

48. **Recognized causes of urticaria include**

    (a) salicylates
    (b) food additives
    (c) systemic lupus erythematosus
    (d) skin sensitivity to pressure
    (e) C_1-esterase inhibitor deficiency

49. **Vitiligo**

    (a) shows familial clustering
    (b) is less common in dark-skinned races
    (c) is associated with Addison's disease
    (d) demonstrates Köebner's phenomenon
    (e) shows anaesthesia in the hypopigmented macules

50. **'Necrobiosis' is a characteristic histopathological feature of the following**

    (a) psoriasis
    (b) rheumatoid nodules
    (c) eczema
    (d) granuloma annulare
    (e) granuloma multiforme

51. **The following are recognized adverse effects of topical steroids**

    (a) telangiectasia
    (b) tinea incognito
    (c) peri-oral dermatitis
    (d) Wickham's striae
    (e) xeroderma pigmentosum

52. **The following associations are correct**

    (a) koilonychia — Mg^{2+} deficiency
    (b) Beau's lines — pneumonia
    (c) paronychia congenita — sex-linked inheritance
    (d) yellow nails — chloroquine therapy
    (e) blue–black discoloration of the nail beds — steroids

53. **Side effects of systemic retinoids include**

    (a) cheilitis
    (b) bony exostosis
    (c) teratogenicity
    (d) epistaxis
    (e) pyogenic granuloma-like lesions on the trunk

54. **The following are characterized by subepidermal blisters**
    (a) pemphigus vulgaris
    (b) erythema multiforme
    (c) burns
    (d) herpes zoster
    (e) porphyria cutanea tarda

55. **Bowen's carcinoma *in situ***
    (a) can be confused clinically with psoriasis
    (b) is related to arsenic ingestion
    (c) develops into metastasizing squamous cell carcinoma in most untreated cases
    (d) typically occurs on sun-exposed areas
    (e) is best treated with cryotherapy

56. **Mycosis fungoides**
    (a) is a B-cell lymphoma involving the skin
    (b) is a recognized cause of erythroderma
    (c) is common
    (d) at presentation, the disease is usually advanced and localized
    (e) is a blistering disease

57. **The clinical features of yaws include**
    (a) plantar hyperkeratosis
    (b) tabes dorsalis
    (c) bone destruction
    (d) positive syphilis serology
    (e) aortitis

58. **The following disorders are found predominantly in childhood**
    (a) psoriasis
    (b) papular urticaria
    (c) epidermolysis bullosa simplex
    (d) staphylococcal scalded skin syndrome
    (e) pityriasis rosea

59. **Lichen planus**
    (a) may affect the genitalia
    (b) accounts for 10% of dermatological outpatients in the UK
    (c) does not respond to steroids
    (d) is characterized by pruritus
    (e) usually resolves spontaneously within a period of 3 months

60. **Rosacea**
    (a) is more common in males
    (b) is best treated by potent topical steroids
    (c) is characterized by comedones
    (d) can be complicated by rhinophyma
    (e) can lead to visual impairment

61. **Psoriatic arthropathy**
    (a) is commonest in Japan
    (b) is a sero-negative arthropathy
    (c) usually spares the terminal interphalangeal joints
    (d) may take the form of arthritis mutilans
    (e) is successfully treated with chloroquine

62. **Abnormal nails may be found in**
    (a) eczema
    (b) icthyosis
    (c) lichen planus
    (d) myxoedema
    (e) Plummer–Vinson syndrome

63. **The causes of penile ulcers include**
    (a) lymphogranuloma venereum
    (b) chancroid
    (c) loiasis
    (d) onchocerciasis
    (e) granuloma inguinale

64. **The following are helpful in the treatment of discoid lupus erythematosus**
    (a) topical hydrocortisone
    (b) sun-light
    (c) hydroxychloroquine sulphate
    (d) oral tetracycline
    (e) camouflaging creams

65. **Pregnancy is associated with**
    (a) herpes gestationis
    (b) frontal alopecia
    (c) erythema marginatum
    (d) lichen planus
    (e) chloasma

66. **Tinea unguium**
   (a) is most commonly due to *Candida albicans*
   (b) is usually associated with nail-pitting
   (c) is a recognized cause of onycholysis
   (d) usually presents with a patch of yellow/white discolouration at the free edge of the nail plate
   (e) is best treated with oral griseofulvin

67. **Paget's disease of the nipple**
   (a) was described by Sir James Paget in 1774
   (b) is always associated with intraduct carcinoma
   (c) can be clinically confused with eczema
   (d) has an excellent prognosis in the absence of a palpable mass
   (e) is commoner in females with Paget's disease of bone

68. **The following skin lesions are due to *Mycobacterium tuberculosis***
   (a) tuberculoid leprosy
   (b) lupus vulgaris
   (c) erythema induratum
   (d) tripe palm
   (e) tuberculosis verrucosa

69. **The following are usually due to staphylococci**
   (a) erysipeloid
   (b) follicular impetigo
   (c) sycosis barbae
   (d) erythrasma
   (e) pityriasis rosea

70. **Anogenital pruritus is seen in**
   (a) thread worm infestation
   (b) *Trichomonas vaginalis* infection
   (c) urinary tract infection
   (d) Parinaud's syndrome
   (e) diabetes mellitus

71. **Clotrimazole**
   (a) increases permeability of fungal membrane
   (b) can be given IV
   (c) is hepatotoxic if given systemically
   (d) is effective against vulval candidiasis
   (e) does not cause local irritation

72. **Topical corticosteroids are effective in**
    - (a) rosacea
    - (b) pityriasis versicolor
    - (c) cold sores
    - (d) athlete's foot
    - (e) molluscum contagiosum

73. **The following parasites affect the skin**
    - (a) *Entamoeba histolytica*
    - (b) *Strongyloides stercoralis*
    - (c) *Wuchereria bancrofti*
    - (d) *Dracunculus medinensis*
    - (e) *Toxocara canis*

74. **Dermographism**
    - (a) occurs in 5% of the population
    - (b) is usually asymptomatic
    - (c) is an exaggerated form of triple response
    - (d) is much more common in patients with urticaria
    - (e) sometimes gives positive transfer tests (when patient's serum is injected into a normal subject)

75. **The following are features of sarcoidosis**
    - (a) lupus vulgaris
    - (b) syringoma
    - (c) erythema nodosum
    - (d) erythrasma
    - (e) miliaria

76. **Herpes simplex is associated with**
    - (a) erythema multiforme
    - (b) hand, foot and mouth disease
    - (c) condyloma acuminatum
    - (d) Kaposi's varicelliform eruption
    - (e) Ramsay Hunt syndrome

77. **Erythroderma is associated with**
    - (a) oliguria
    - (b) lymphadenopathy
    - (c) anaemia
    - (d) gynaecomastia
    - (e) hypocalcaemia

78. **Hyperhidrosis is a feature of**

   (a) acromegaly
   (b) tuberculosis
   (c) miliaria
   (d) prematurity
   (e) psoriasis

79. **Hypertrichosis is a feature of**

   (a) dermatomyositis
   (b) porphyria cutanea tarda
   (c) diazoxide therapy
   (d) malnutrition in childhood
   (e) anorexia nervosa

80. **Patchy hypopigmentation of the skin is a feature of**

   (a) neurofibromatosis
   (b) Peutz-Jeghers disease
   (c) pityriasis versicolor
   (d) pityriasis alba
   (e) leprosy

81. **Generalized hyperpigmentation is a feature of**

   (a) hypopituitarism
   (b) primary hypoadrenalism
   (c) carcinoma
   (d) phenylketonuria
   (e) acanthosis nigricans

82. **Wood's light**

   (a) emits short-wave UVR
   (b) fluoresces lesions due to *Microsporum canis* yellow
   (c) shows yellow fluorescence with *Malassezia furfur*
   (d) fluoresces lesions due to *Corynebacterium minutissimum* coral red
   (e) shows coral pink fluorescence with urine from porphyria cutanea tarda patients

83. **Darier's disease**

   (a) is transmitted by autosomal recessive inheritance
   (b) commonly presents as greasy brown papules on the chest
   (c) affects the nails
   (d) is treated with retinoid etretinate given systemically in severe cases
   (e) is improved by sunlight

84. **The following are features of Ehlers–Danlos syndrome**
    (a) autosomal dominant inheritance in all biochemical variants
    (b) muscular hypertonia
    (c) hernia formation
    (d) dissecting aneurysms
    (e) lax skin

85. **Features of secondary syphilis include**
    (a) tabes dorsalis
    (b) condyloma latum
    (c) snail-track ulcers
    (d) gumma
    (e) lymphadenopathy

86. **The following skin diseases are helped by sunlight**
    (a) lupus erythromatosus
    (b) eczema
    (c) venous leg ulcers
    (d) psoriasis
    (e) porphyria cutanea tarda

87. **The following cutaneous manifestations are associated with carcinoma of the pancreas**
    (a) pruritus
    (b) nodular panniculitis
    (c) superficial thrombophlebitis
    (d) erythema multiforme
    (e) pemphigus vulgaris

88. **Progressive systemic sclerosis**
    (a) typically presents after the age of 60 years
    (b) is associated with primary biliary sclerosis
    (c) has an overall 5 year survival of 10%
    (d) is more common than SLE
    (e) affects the gastrointestinal tract in the majority of cases

89. **Induration of the skin may be a feature of**
    (a) acromegaly
    (b) amyloidosis
    (c) scleroderma
    (d) scleromyxoedema
    (e) steroid therapy

90. **Acne can be induced by**

   (a) ACTH
   (b) cough mixtures
   (c) cosmetics
   (d) exposure to small amounts of chlorphenols
   (e) clindamycin topical solution

91. **Drug eruptions**

   (a) are always fixed 'l'éruption fixé'
   (b) are mostly due to the development of hypersensitivity
   (c) sometimes show cross-sensitization
   (d) always clear within two weeks after stopping the drug
   (e) are usually accompanied by pyrexia

92. **Causes of finger clubbing include**

   (a) bronchiectasis
   (b) thyrotoxicosis
   (c) iron deficiency
   (d) psoriasis
   (e) bacterial endocarditis

93. **The following are examples of exogenous eczema**

   (a) gravitational eczema
   (b) discoid eczema
   (c) contact dermatitis
   (d) pompholyx
   (e) seborrhoeic dermatitis

94. **Flushing is a feature of**

   (a) dumping syndrome
   (b) carcinoid syndrome
   (c) adrenalectomy
   (d) verapamil therapy
   (e) rosacea

95. **Premature greying of hair is increased in**

   (a) pernicious anaemia
   (b) medical students
   (c) Graves' disease
   (d) Albright's syndrome
   (e) Waardenburg's syndrome

96. **Neuropathic ulcers are particularly associated with**
(a) porphyria
(b) amyloidosis
(c) leprosy
(d) tabes dorsalis
(e) diabetes mellitus

97. **Telogen effluvium**
(a) the heavy and rapid hair loss usually occurs 1–2 weeks after a stressful event
(b) is best treated with oral steroids
(c) is characterized by broken hairs that resemble exclamation marks
(d) may be associated with Beau's lines on the nails
(e) spontaneous regrowth of hair usually occurs within the next 6 months

98. **Pellagra is a recognized feature of**
(a) tryptophan therapy for depression
(b) carcinoid syndrome
(c) high protein diets
(d) Hartnup disease
(e) isoniazid therapy

99. **Surgical excision is the treatment of choice in**
(a) Kaposi's sarcoma
(b) Bowen's disease
(c) basal cell carcinoma
(d) glomus tumour
(e) port wine stain

100. **The following are true about psoriasis**
(a) the commonest age of presentation is in the fifth decade
(b) it is associated with HLA-Cw6
(c) the guttate form is commoner in adults than in children
(d) flexor aspects of knees are commonest sites of involvement
(e) it is premalignant

101. **Bullous pemphigoid**
(a) is commoner in the Jewish race
(b) is treated with systemic steroids
(c) may affect the oral cavity
(d) is characterized by intra-epidermal blisters
(e) presents with large tense blisters mainly on the back

102. **Pyogenic granuloma**
   (a) is due to *Bacillus anthracis*
   (b) develops after trauma
   (c) is highly vascular
   (d) is associated with diabetes mellitus
   (e) is treated with systemic antibiotics

103. **Purpura is a feature of**
   (a) Cushing's syndrome
   (b) thrombocytopenia
   (c) Wiskott–Aldrich syndrome
   (d) meningococcal septicaemia
   (e) vasculitis

104. **Lichen simplex**
   (a) is commoner in men
   (b) is due to external irritants
   (c) is associated with atopy
   (d) is characterized by itch–scratch–itch cycle
   (e) responds to systemic steroids best

105. **Lupus vulgaris**
   (a) is most common in the tropics
   (b) is treated with anti-tuberculous drugs
   (c) affects males more often than females
   (d) most commonly affects the face and neck
   (e) is premalignant

106. **The following disorders and causatives are correctly paired**
   (a) Buruli ulcer — *Borrelia recurrentis*
   (b) swimming pool granuloma — *Mycobacterium ulcerans*
   (c) creeping eruption — *Onchocerca volvulus*
   (d) epidermolysis bullosa — staphylococci
   (e) Stevens–Johnson syndrome — long acting sulphonamides

107. **Sarcoidosis**
   (a) may present with anterior uveitis
   (b) is associated with a strongly positive Mantoux test
   (c) can be confused clinically with beryllium poisoning
   (d) does not affect the bone
   (e) erythema induratum is the commonest dermatological presentation

108. **The following are clinical features of Reiter's disease**
   (a) keratoderma blenorrhagica
   (b) erosive arthritis
   (c) Lowe's syndrome
   (d) low back pain
   (e) circinate balanitis

109. **Molluscum contagiosum**
   (a) lesions never affect the face
   (b) atopic individuals are particularly prone to infection
   (c) demonstrates Köebner's phenomenon
   (d) biopsy is usually required to make the diagnosis
   (e) is caused by a pox virus

110. **Pityriasis rubra pilaris**
   (a) may affect the scalp
   (b) can be confused clinically with psoriasis
   (c) gives a positive Wasserman reaction (WR) test
   (d) is caused by a fungus
   (e) usually, resolves spontaneously over 6 days

111. **Clinical features of primary herpes simplex include**
   (a) keratoconjunctivitis
   (b) difficulty in swallowing
   (c) vulvovaginitis
   (d) encephalitis
   (e) neuralgia

112. **The following are useful measures in the management of atopic eczema in children**
   (a) emollients
   (b) 1% hydrocortisone
   (c) wool underclothes to keep the child warm
   (d) salicylic acid
   (e) tying the hands to prevent scratching

113. **The following are inherited in an X-linked fashion**
   (a) ataxia-telangiectasia
   (b) Menkes disease
   (c) hypohidrotic ectodermal dysplasia
   (d) xeroderma pigmentosum
   (e) erythropoietic porphyrias

114. **The dermatological features of kwashiorkor include**
   (a) cracked skin
   (b) hair-thickening
   (c) skin atrophy
   (d) petechial macules
   (e) moon facies

115. **Dupuytren's contracture**
   (a) is associated with epilepsy
   (b) there is a higher incidence in diabetes mellitus
   (c) fasciectomy is the treatment of choice
   (d) is common before the age of 30 years
   (e) is always unilateral

116. **The adult worm of the following is located in the skin**
   (a) *Wuchereria bancrofti*
   (b) *loa loa*
   (c) *Onchocerca volvulus*
   (d) *Brugia malayi*
   (e) *Trichinella spiralis*

117. **Indications for use of intralesional corticosteroids include**
   (a) acne cysts
   (b) granuloma annulare
   (c) orf
   (d) hypertrophic lichen planus
   (e) necrobiosis lipoidica

118. **The following are useful in the management of epidermolysis bullosa**
   (a) plastic surgery
   (b) occupational therapy
   (c) radiotherapy
   (d) coal tar
   (e) genetic counselling

119. **The clinical features of polymyositis/dermatomyositis complex include**
   (a) low levels of creatine phosphokinase in serum
   (b) polyarthritis
   (c) waddling gait
   (d) Nikolsky's sign
   (e) a heliotrope rash around the eyes

120. **Clinical features of systemic lupus erythematosus include**

    (a) loss of hair
    (b) Raynaud's phenomenon
    (c) telangiectasia at the base of the nail
    (d) photosensitivity
    (e) subcutaneous nodules

121. **Clinical features of acrodermatitis enteropathica include**

    (a) diarrhoea
    (b) high serum zinc
    (c) pustules
    (d) pyoderma gangrenosum
    (e) granuloma annulare

122. **The differential diagnosis of tinea pedis includes**

    (a) simple maceration of the skin
    (b) excessive sweating
    (c) pityriasis rosea
    (d) eczema
    (e) psoriasis

123. **Keloids**

    (a) are, most commonly, caused by surgery
    (b) may follow a viral infection of the dermis
    (c) are commoner in caucasians
    (d) are characterized by abnormal epidermis
    (e) never form spontaneously

124. **Linear lesions are a feature of**

    (a) pityriasis rosea
    (b) viral warts
    (c) psoriasis
    (d) lichen planus
    (e) erythema annulare

125. **Annular lesions are a feature of**

    (a) creeping eruption
    (b) tinea corporis
    (c) pityriasis rosea
    (d) partially treated psoriasis
    (e) urticaria

126. **The following are effective in the treatment of viral warts**
    (a) curettage and cautery
    (b) podophyllin
    (c) carbon dioxide snow
    (d) intralesional steroids
    (e) systemic acyclovir

127. **The following are common blistering eruptions**
    (a) epidermolysis bullosa
    (b) scabies
    (c) herpes zoster
    (d) incontinentia pigmenti
    (e) pompholyx

128. **Pediculosis capitis**
    (a) may present with impetigo
    (b) is characterized by nits on the hair shaft
    (c) affects the trunk
    (d) is contagious
    (e) is effectively treated with the application of 1% solution of benzene-hexachloride after the hair has been washed

129. **Potent topical steroids include**
    (a) clobetasol propionate 0.05%
    (b) hydrocortisone (1%)
    (c) clobetasone butyrate 0.05%
    (d) methylprednisolone 0.25%
    (e) beclomethasone dipropionate 0.5%

130. **The following dermatoses usually have a symmetrical distribution**
    (a) impetigo
    (b) tinea corporis
    (c) vitiligo
    (d) lichen planus
    (e) exogenous eczema

131. **Systemic griseofulvin is effective against**
    (a) dermatophyte infection
    (b) pityriasis versicolor
    (c) erysipelas
    (d) *Taenia solium*
    (e) *Candida* infection

132. **The following eruptions are characteristically centrifugal**
   (a) chicken pox
   (b) pityriasis rosea
   (c) rosacea
   (d) shagreen patches
   (e) erythema multiforme

133. **Peyronie's disease**
   (a) is a recognized feature of sarcoidosis
   (b) may resolve spontaneously
   (c) does not result in impotence
   (d) is due to over-production of collagen
   (e) is associated with Dupuytren's contractures

134. **Discoid eczema**
   (a) usually affects children
   (b) is characterized by circular lesions ranging from 4mm to 10mm in diameter
   (c) is an example of endogenous eczema
   (d) is effectively controlled with topical steroids
   (e) is always associated with pruritus

135. **Chicken pox**
   (a) spreads by droplet infection from infectious patients
   (b) can spread transplacentally
   (c) is associated with Koplik's spots in the buccal mucosa
   (d) the rash consists of vesicles all of which appear simultaneously
   (e) cannot be acquired by contact with cases of shingles

136. **Kaposi's sarcoma**
   (a) usually spares the indigenous black population in Africa
   (b) is associated with HLA-DR5
   (c) is commonly found in the brains of affected AIDS patients
   (d) can be clinically confused with pyogenic granuloma
   (e) histologically consists of spindle-cells with vascular elements

137. **The following cutaneous diseases occur in the male genital skin**
   (a) lichen planus
   (b) atopic dermatitis
   (c) erythema multiforme
   (d) molluscum contagiosum
   (e) Peyronie's disease

138. **Dermatoglyphic ridge patterns**
    (a) change throughout life
    (b) are unique to every individual
    (c) are diagnostically useful in some congenital diseases
    (d) are arranged in triradii only
    (e) can be influenced by drugs in the early fetal life

139. **Indications for PUVA therapy include**
    (a) mycosis fungoides
    (b) resistant chronic pompholyx
    (c) porphyria cutanea tarda
    (d) psoriasis
    (e) xeroderma pigmentosum

140. **First degree burns**
    (a) are characterized by blisters
    (b) involve the upper dermis
    (c) heal with scarring
    (d) are painful and hypersensitive
    (e) take 4 weeks to heal

141. **Intra-oral lesions are present in the following infections**
    (a) rubella
    (b) smallpox
    (c) moniliasis
    (d) herpes simplex
    (e) herpangina

142. **Chancroid**
    (a) presents with genital ulcers
    (b) is best treated with intramuscular penicillin
    (c) is more common in women
    (d) does not usually affect the mouth
    (e) is followed by long-standing immunity

143. **Cutaneous manifestations of immunodeficiency include**
    (a) folliculitis
    (b) seborrhoeic dermatitis
    (c) graft-versus-host reaction
    (d) chronic mucocutaneous candidiasis
    (e) skin cancer

144. **Causes of necrosis of the skin include**
    (a) cryoglobinaemia
    (b) intravenous bleomycin
    (c) anthrax
    (d) electric energy
    (e) syphilis

145. **The following disorders are associated with acanthosis**
    (a) psoriasis
    (b) lichen planus
    (c) pityriasis rosea
    (d) Reiter's syndrome
    (e) ichthyosis

146. **The clinical features of pseudoxanthoma elasticum include**
    (a) loose skin over neck, axillae and groins
    (b) hypotension in 50% of cases
    (c) claudication
    (d) thyrotoxicosis
    (e) plucked chicken-skin appearance

147. **Acanthosis nigricans is associated with**
    (a) Cushing's syndrome
    (b) gastric adenocarcinoma
    (c) Stein–Leventhal syndrome
    (d) bronchial carcinoma
    (e) candidiasis

148. **Arterial spiders (spider naevi)**
    (a) are common in pregnancy
    (b) are most frequently seen on the lower extremities
    (c) when solitary, strongly suggest hepatic cirrhosis
    (d) are true tumours of cutaneous arteries
    (e) may be treated with cautery

149. **Exudation of serum (weeping) is a feature of**
    (a) eczema
    (b) ichthyosis vulgaris
    (c) vitiligo
    (d) tuberculoid leprosy
    (e) the primary chancre of syphyilis

150. **The differential diagnosis of tinea corporis includes**
    (a) psoriasis
    (b) impetigo
    (c) pityriasis rosea
    (d) erythema nodosum
    (e) adenoma sebaceum

151. **The following forms of cutaneous leishmaniasis are typically found in the Mediterranean, USSR and India**
    (a) chiclero ulcer
    (b) diffuse cutaneous leishmaniasis
    (c) leishmaniasis tropica minor
    (d) espundia (mucocutaneous leishmaniasis)
    (e) uta

152. **Atopic eczema**
    (a) affects 3% of children
    (b) is often associated with positive skin prick tests
    (c) is a contra-indication to immunization against diphtheria
    (d) is more common in breast feeding rather than cow's milk feeding
    (e) ensures a form of immunity against infection with herpes simplex

153. **Carcinoma of the penis**
    (a) is commoner in the Jewish race
    (b) is usually seen in males aged 25–34 years
    (c) may be precipitated by human papilloma virus
    (d) has a five-year survival rate of 65% if treated with radiotherapy
    (e) the lymph nodes in the groin are enlarged in 10% of cases

154. **Variegate porphyria**
    (a) is associated with hepatocellular carcinoma
    (b) the main abnormality lies in the enzyme uroporphyrinogen decarboxylase
    (c) is not associated with cutaneous manifestations
    (d) is classified as an erythropoietic porphyria
    (e) the usual onset is in infancy

155. **The clinical features of polyarteritis nodosa include**
    (a) granuloma annulare
    (b) females are more frequently affected
    (c) an association with hepatitis B virus surface antigen
    (d) Thibierge–Weissenbach syndrome
    (e) peripheral neuropathy

156. **Causes of palmar erythema include**
   (a) thyrotoxicosis
   (b) alcoholic cirrhosis
   (c) polycythaemia
   (d) pregnancy
   (e) shoulder−hand syndrome

157. **The following cause conjunctivitis with oral and genital ulcers**
   (a) Anton's syndrome
   (b) Stevens−Johnson syndrome
   (c) Behcet's syndrome
   (d) pityriasis versicolor
   (e) Reiter's syndrome

158. **Porphyria cutanea tarda**
   (a) is associated with low serum iron
   (b) is associated with hepatocellular carcinoma
   (c) most patients are over 60 years
   (d) patients may develop haemorrhage blisters on light-exposure
   (e) recurrence is reduced by avoiding alcohol

159. **Gianotti−Crosti syndrome**
   (a) is commonest in the elderly
   (b) is chiefly localized to the extremities
   (c) is helped by topical steroids
   (d) is intensely itchy
   (e) spontaneously heals in about 6 weeks

160. **The differential diagnosis of vitiligo includes**
   (a) leprosy
   (b) pityriasis versicolor
   (c) albinism
   (d) dermatitis herpetiformis
   (e) lentigo maligna

161. **The following typically present after the age of 50 years**
   (a) dermatitis herpetiformis
   (b) psoriasis
   (c) bullous pemphigoid
   (d) alopecia areata
   (e) Bowen's disease

162. **Erythema multiforme**
 (a) usually affects the elderly
 (b) is commonly triggered by herpes simplex infection
 (c) is a recognized cause of corneal ulceration
 (d) may be precipitated by chlorpropamide
 (e) principally affects the trunk

163. **Venous ulceration**
 (a) is never malignant
 (b) typically occurs on the medial side of the lower leg
 (c) is usually due to venous stasis
 (d) is more common in males
 (e) can be prevented by supportive stockings after a deep venous thrombosis

164. **Carcinoma of the lip**
 (a) usually affects the lower lip
 (b) is more common in females
 (c) is associated with pipe smoking
 (d) usually presents as an enlarging chronic ulcer
 (e) is adenocarcinoma in most cases

165. **Erysipelas**
 (a) is usually caused by staphylococci
 (b) may be mimicked by rosacea
 (c) is best treated by topical antibiotics
 (d) is less serious than impetigo
 (e) is commonest on the face and legs

166. **The differential diagnosis of a primary chancre includes**
 (a) herpes simplex
 (b) chancroid
 (c) Peyronie's disease of the penis
 (d) erosive balanitis
 (e) squamous cell carcinoma of the penis

167. **Granuloma annulare**
 (a) heals spontaneously without scarring
 (b) usually presents as flesh-coloured papules on the back of the hands
 (c) responds to antibiotics
 (d) predominantly affects the elderly
 (e) may be confused with sarcoidosis

168. **Peri-anal warts**
    (a) are due to a rota virus
    (b) are more common in homosexual men
    (c) never extend into the rectum
    (d) are common in children
    (e) are also known as condyloma acuminatum

169. **Primary irritant dermatitis**
    (a) has atopy as a predisposing feature
    (b) is usually due to a previous exposure to allergen
    (c) relies upon patch testing to identify the irritant
    (d) may be helped by topical steroids
    (e) is common among housewives

170. **Pilonidal sinus**
    (a) is more common in females
    (b) most commonly affects the natal clefts
    (c) usually presents with a history of recurrent abcesses
    (d) is best treated conservatively with antibiotics
    (e) is common in children

171. **The cutaneous manifestations of pancreatitis include**
    (a) café-au-lait patches
    (b) a Herald patch
    (c) Cullen's sign
    (d) Grey Turner's sign
    (e) jaundice

172. **The clinical features of Lyme disease include**
    (a) myocarditis
    (b) erythema chronicum migrans
    (c) von Hippel–Lindau syndrome
    (d) fever
    (e) arthritis

173. **The following have a malignant potential**
    (a) port wine haemangioma
    (b) cavernous lymphangioma
    (c) dermoid cyst
    (d) lipoma
    (e) intradermal naevus

174. **The following are features of secondary syphilis**
   (a) gumma
   (b) Argyll Robertson pupil
   (c) a negative Wasserman reaction (WR) test
   (d) condyloma latum
   (e) patchy hair loss

175. **Alopecia areata**
   (a) has a lower incidence among atopic subjects
   (b) accounts for about 2% of dermatological out-patient attendances in the UK and USA
   (c) usually follows a systemic insult
   (d) is associated with vitiligo in about 4% of cases
   (e) never progresses to alopecia totalis

176. **The following are helpful in treating discoid lupus erythematosus**
   (a) sunlight
   (b) topical steroids
   (c) antibiotics
   (d) hydroxychloroquine
   (e) cosmetic creams

177. **A honeycomb lung is a recognized feature of**
   (a) neurofibromatosis
   (b) sarcoidosis
   (c) tuberose sclerosis
   (d) trichitillomania
   (e) systemic sclerosis

178. **Sarcoidosis**
   (a) is the commonest cause of erythema nodosum
   (b) affects the skin in 60% of cases
   (c) is a cause of painful red eye
   (d) is commonly complicated by hypocalcaemia
   (e) carries a better prognosis in black races

179. **Hutchinson's summer prurigo**
   (a) is a complication of congenital syphilis
   (b) usually presents with erythema and blisters rather than papules on sun-exposed areas
   (c) does not always clear in the winter
   (d) has been reported to respond to thalidomide
   (e) is usually seen in children

180. **The differential diagnosis of palmar tinea includes**
   (a) pityriasis rosea
   (b) contact dermatitis
   (c) rosacea
   (d) snail track ulcers
   (e) psoriasis

181. **Eosinophilia is a feature of**
   (a) scabies
   (b) dermatitis herpetiformis
   (c) urticaria
   (d) eczema
   (e) Hodgkin's disease

182. **The following topical therapies are useful in rosacea**
   (a) topical 5-fluorouracil (5FU)
   (b) 0.05% clobetasol propionate
   (c) metronidazole
   (d) sulphur cream
   (e) clotrimazole solution

183. **Causes of mouth ulcers include**
   (a) methotrexate
   (b) herpes simplex
   (c) squamous cell carcinoma
   (d) syphilis
   (e) pemphigus vulgaris

184. **The following are common causes of a pigmented papule**
   (a) acute intermittent porphyria
   (b) basal cell papilloma
   (c) dermatofibroma
   (d) melanocytic naevus
   (e) Nelson's syndrome

185. **Most patients with infective endocarditis have**
    (a) Osler nodes
    (b) clubbing
    (c) Janeway lesions
    (d) cardiac murmurs
    (e) splinter haemorrhages

186. **The following are helpful in seborrhoeic dermatitis**
    (a) selenium sulphide in a shampoo form
    (b) oral steroids
    (c) dithranol
    (d) topical minoxidil
    (e) 2 month course of low dose tetracycline

187. **Ingrowing toe-nail**
    (a) is common before the age of 5 years
    (b) has a familial predisposition
    (c) usually affects the big toe
    (d) is always treated surgically
    (e) may recur after treatment by Zadek's operation

188. **Causes of purpura include**
    (a) eczema
    (b) senility
    (c) meningococcaemia
    (d) steroids
    (e) vasculitis

189. **Juvenile plantar dermatosis**
    (a) responds well to steroid ointments
    (b) is commonest after puberty
    (c) improves with wearing permeable leather shoes
    (d) was very common in the 1950s
    (e) is characterized by a scaly fissured erythema on the fore-foot

190. **Tuberculoid leprosy**
    (a) shows a very weak type IV hypersensitivity reaction to lepromin
    (b) is due to *Mycobacterium tuberculosis*
    (c) shows many bacilli in the skin smears
    (d) usually presents with an anaesthetic hypopigmented macule
    (e) is associated with hypertrichosis at the site of lesion

191. The following are pathological features of psoriasis
    (a) acanthosis
    (b) hypokeratosis
    (c) increased epidermal transit time
    (d) elongated rete ridges
    (e) epidermal micro-abcesses

192. The following are cutaneous manifestations of underlying malignancy
    (a) pallor
    (b) flushing
    (c) herpes zoster
    (d) psoriasis
    (e) lichen planus

193. Periungual erythema is a sign of
    (a) syringoma
    (b) tuberculoid leprosy
    (c) lupus erythromatosus
    (d) systemic sclerosis
    (e) dermatomyositis

194. The following words and statements are correctly paired
    (a) crust — a flake of keratin
    (b) ecchymosis — a small purpuric lesion
    (c) macule — a small raised area
    (d) vesicle — a small blister
    (e) telengiectasia — permanently dilated visible small vessels

195. The histological features of eczema include
    (a) follicular plugging
    (b) parakeratosis
    (c) constriction of dermal blood vessels
    (d) hyperkeratosis
    (e) dermal infiltration by lymphocytes

196. Arsenic ingestion is associated with
    (a) ichthyosis erythroderma
    (b) Bowen's disease
    (c) small circular brown keratoses on the palms and soles
    (d) psoriasis
    (e) lichen simplex

197. **Indications for etretinate include**

(a) pustular psoriasis during pregnancy
(b) severe Darier's disease
(c) congenital ichthyosis
(d) paronychia
(e) alopecia

198. **The cutaneous complications of diabetes mellitus include**

(a) acquired ichthyosis
(b) bullae
(c) pruritus vulvae
(d) brown scars over the shins
(e) mucocutaneous candidiasis

199. **The following are recognized complications of sebaceous cysts**

(a) keratoacanthoma (molluscum sebaceum)
(b) calcification
(c) horn formation
(d) ulceration
(e) infection

200. **Hereditary angio-oedema**

(a) has an autosomal recessive inheritance
(b) is due to deficiency of C1q part of the complement system
(c) can be fatal
(d) is a cause of urticaria
(e) may present as an acute abdomen

201. **The following dermatoses may worsen during pregnancy**

(a) rosacea
(b) acne
(c) eczema
(d) candidiasis
(e) psoriasis

202. **Topical steroids help**

(a) peri-oral dermatitis
(b) most types of psoriasis
(c) rosacea
(d) striae of the skin
(e) tinea cruris

203. **The following are birth marks**

    (a) cradle cap
    (b) Casal's necklace
    (c) strawberry naevus
    (d) port wine stain
    (e) Beau's lines

204. **Yellow discoloration of nails is a feature of**

    (a) antimalarial therapy
    (b) pustular psoriasis
    (c) dermatophyte infections
    (d) hypoalbuminaemia
    (e) phenothiazine administration

205. **The following are biological features of old age**

    (a) senile sebaceous atrophy
    (b) dry skin
    (c) impaired wound healing
    (d) peripheral ischaemia
    (e) increased sweating

206. **Macular amyloidosis**

    (a) is a characteristic feature of systemic amyloidosis
    (b) is less common in Asians
    (c) is synonymous with lichen amyloidosis
    (d) commonly affects shoulders, neck and upper back
    (e) it is difficult to demonstrate the amyloid using routine histological methods

207. **The following are related to sports**

    (a) otitis externa
    (b) Vogt–Koyanagi–Harada syndrome
    (c) Von Zumbusch syndrome
    (d) chilblains
    (e) miliaria

208. **The following are sexually transmited**

    (a) molluscum contagiosum
    (b) vaginal candidiasis
    (c) scabies
    (d) Rieter's disease
    (e) Forrestier's disease (ankylosing vertebral hyperostosis)

209. **The following are recognized causes of erythroderma**
    (a) pityriasis rubra pilaris
    (b) seborrhoeic dermatitis in the elderly
    (c) mycosis fungoides
    (d) morphia
    (e) Kugelberg–Welander disease

210. **Pyogenic granuloma**
    (a) is pus-forming
    (b) is due to granulomatous inflammation
    (c) is often due to trauma
    (d) has malignant melanoma as a differential diagnosis
    (e) is best treated with curettage and diathermy

211. **Orf**
    (a) is caused by an echovirus
    (b) is a recognized cause of erythema multiforme
    (c) lesions usually settle in 10 days
    (d) is synonymous with milker's nodes
    (e) is usually followed by life-long immunity

212. **CNS-involvement is a recognized feature of the following dermatoses**
    (a) Sjögren–Larsson syndrome
    (b) epidermal naevus syndrome
    (c) Campbell de Morgan spots
    (d) tuberous sclerosis
    (e) Sturge–Weber syndrome

213. **The following are recognized causes of nappy rash**
    (a) diarrhoea
    (b) milia
    (c) seborrhoeic dermatitis
    (d) contact dermatitis
    (e) rubeosis

214. **The clinical features of chronic arterial ischaemia of the legs include**
    (a) varicose ulcers
    (b) hairless skin over the legs
    (c) intermittent claudication
    (d) painful punched-out ulcers
    (e) thickened toe-nails

215. **The kidney and skin may be simultaneously involved in the following**
    (a) amyloidosis
    (b) polyarteritis nodosa
    (c) Hartnup disease
    (d) tuberous sclerosis
    (e) rheumatoid arthritis

216. **The clinical features of McCune–Albright syndrome include**
    (a) pathological fractures
    (b) sexual precosity in females
    (c) a positive Mitsuda reaction
    (d) 'café-au-lait' spots
    (e) an association with hyperparathyroidism

217. **The lung and skin may be simultaneously involved in**
    (a) Churg–Strauss syndrome
    (b) sulphonamide therapy
    (c) bronchial carcinoma
    (d) tuberous sclerosis
    (e) histiocytosis X

218. **Urticaria pigmentosa**
    (a) is commoner in adults
    (b) responds well to aspirin
    (c) is characterized by pigmented lesions widely distributed on the trunk
    (d) is an example of mastocytosis
    (e) has a better prognosis in the adult

219. **Systemic steroids are effective in**
    (a) erythema multiforme in children
    (b) aggressive pyoderma gangrenosum
    (c) pemphigus vulgaris
    (d) erysipeloid
    (e) severe acne

220. **The clinical features of Marfan's syndrome include**
    (a) aortic stenosis
    (b) Steinberg's sign
    (c) striae distensae
    (d) Holmes–Adie pupil
    (e) long thin digits

The Answers

1. (a) T
   (b) T
   (c) F the soles are affected; it is seen in 10% of patients with Reiter's syndrome
   (d) T
   (e) F the fingers, the palms, the toes and soles are affected with vesicular rash
2. (a) F the associated malabsorption is usually mild and gastrointestinal symptoms are rare
   (b) T
   (c) T Dapsone (or sulphapyridine) also helps to control the rash
   (d) T
   (e) F
3. (a) T
   (b) T
   (c) T
   (d) F this is a syndrome of intestinal adenomatosis with mesodermal tumours
   (e) T
4. (a) T
   (b) T neuropathic ulcers
   (c) F P. amiantacea is a scalp condition with large silvery scales
   (d) T due to vasculitis
   (e) T pyoderma gangrenosum is a cutaneous manifestation of this disease
5. (a) F the term 'seborrhoeic wart' is misnomer; the sebaceous tissue is not involved
   (b) T
   (c) T
   (d) F
   (e) T
6. (a) T the organism isolated is *Corynebacterium minutissimum*
   (b) F it is not due to a fungus but to diphtheroids
   (c) T
   (d) T
   (e) F systemic flucloxacillin is required; necrotic skin and abcess formation may require surgery
7. (a) F these sites are rarely involved
   (b) T
   (c) F UVR improves the condition
   (d) F secondary syphilis is an important differential diagnosis
   (e) F herald patch precedes the generalized rash by a week or so

8. All **T**

9. (a) **F**
   (b) **F** is associated with hypothyroidism
   (c) **F**
   (d) **T**
   (e) **F**

10. (a) **T** (controversial)
    (b) **F** (this is seen in hypothyroid patients)
    (c) **T**
    (d) **T** due to hyperlipidaemia
    (e) **F** this is a feature of rheumatic fever

11. (a) **T** is a feature of lymphoma
    (b) **T** may be seen in pancreatic malignancy
    (c) **T** is seen in carcinoid syndrome
    (d) **T** pancreatic malignancy (glucagonoma)
    (e) **T**

12. (a) **F** ichthyosis vulgaris is dominantly inherited
    (b) **T**
    (c) **T**
    (d) **F** AIP does not affect the skin
    (e) **T** both conditions are associated with autoimmune diseases

13. (a) **F** the flexures are usually affected
    (b) **T**
    (c) **F** characteristically affect the trunk
    (d) **T**
    (e) **T**

14. (a) **T**
    (b) **T**
    (c) **T**
    (d) **F** skin in rheumatoid arthritis is thin due to loss of collagen
    (e) **T**

15. (a) **T**
    (b) **F** many side effects (e.g. dryness of skin and mucous membranes, alopecia, nausea and vomiting, etc.)
    (c) **F** there is a high risk of teratogenicity
    (d) **T**
    (e) **T**

16.	(a)	T	
	(b)	T	
	(c)	T	
	(d)	T	
	(e)	F	this is carcinoma *in situ* affecting the penis
17.	(a)	T	ichthyosis is seen in 10% of cases
	(b)	F	
	(c)	T	this is the most frequent association
	(d)	F	
	(e)	T	
18.	(a)	T	
	(b)	T	
	(c)	F	AIP does not affect the skin
	(d)	T	
	(e)	T	
19.	(a)	T	
	(b)	T	
	(c)	T	
	(d)	F	commoner in young females
	(e)	F	respond poorly to all treatment modalities including psychiatric intervention
20.	(a)	F	diagnosis is confirmed by biopsy of involved skin
	(b)	F	inflammation only responds (not scarring)
	(c)	T	
	(d)	F	about 5% of cases may progress to SLE
	(e)	T	
21.	(a)	F	the organism isolated is *Corynebacterium minutissimum*
	(b)	F	
	(c)	T	
	(d)	F	responds to oral erythromycin and some topical antibiotics
	(e)	T	
22.	(a)	T	
	(b)	T	
	(c)	T	as in pellagra
	(d)	T	
	(e)	T	

23. (a) T there is hypercholesterolaemia due to increased synthesis
    (b) T this type is characterized by hypercholesterolaemia and normal triglycerides
    (c) T
    (d) T eruptive xanthoma due to hyperlipidaemia are common in diabetes mellitus
    (e) F

24. (a) T
    (b) F
    (c) T
    (d) F
    (e) T

25. (a) F it is a *delusion* of infestation with parasites or insects!
    (b) T
    (c) T
    (d) T
    (e) F the prognosis is poor regardless of whether the patient is treated by a dermatologist or a psychiatrist

26. (a) F should be taken with meals for better absorption
    (b) F it is fungistatic only
    (c) F
    (d) F
    (e) T also contra-indicated in porphyria and severe lung disease

27. (a) T
    (b) T
    (c) T
    (d) F this leads to defective collagen synthesis and abnormal vessel wall with haemorrhage, purpura, anaemia, etc.
    (e) T (hereditary haemorrhagic telengiectasia)

28. (a) F patients are usually middle-aged or elderly
    (b) T
    (c) T
    (d) F disseminated zoster may affect other organs, e.g. meninges, lungs, etc.
    (e) F the motor roots can also be involved

29. (a) F caused by human papilloma viruses which are DNA viruses
    (b) F the hands and knees are usually affected
    (c) T
    (d) T
    (e) T

30. (a) **T**
    (b) **T**
    (c) **T**
    (d) **T**
    (e) **F** this is a Ca^{2+}-channel blocker that causes vasodilation

31. (a) **F** it has a better prognosis in females
    (b) **T**
    (c) **F** this is a poor prognostic sign
    (d) **F**
    (e) **F**

32. (a) **F** in this syndrome the nails and the patellae are hypoplastic or absent
    (b) **T** especially males with diabetes, aged 15–20 years
    (c) **T**
    (d) **F** this may be associated with pitting of the nails
    (e) **F** deficiency of sulphur-containing amino acids as a result of poor nutrition may give rise to this

33. (a) **T**
    (b) **F** the deficient enzyme is usually tyrosinase, whereas lack of phenylalanine-4-hydroxylase is the underlying abnormality in phenylketonuria
    (c) **T** due to lack of protective melanin
    (d) **T** due to failure of melanin synthesis
    (e) **F** autosomal recessive

34. (a) **F** (the human IgG is attached to the intercellular cement of the epidermis)
    (b) **T**
    (c) **T**
    (d) **F** abnormal findings are seen in involved skin only
    (e) **T**

35. All **T**

36. (a) **T**
    (b) **F** there is usually a diffuse hair loss
    (c) **T**
    (d) **F** the hair loss is usually diffuse
    (e) **T** occasionally it may progress to alopecia totalis (the whole scalp) or alopecia universalis (the whole body)

37. All **T**

38. (a) **T**
    (b) **T** if protective glasses are not worn
    (c) **T**
    (d) **F** in fact it may help the condition
    (e) **F**

39. (a) **T**
    (b) **T**
    (c) **F** this is characteristic of pityriasis rosea
    (d) **T** these are angiofibromas
    (e) **T** ash leaf macules

40. (a) **T**
    (b) **T**
    (c) **F** this is a different dermatosis which may be due to a virus
    (d) **F** this is a fungal infection
    (e) **T**

41. (a) **T**
    (b) **F** this is seen in tuberous sclerosis
    (c) **F**
    (d) **T**
    (e) **T** this is the commonest cutaneous manifestation

42. (a) **T**
    (b) **F** Cushing's syndrome is a recognized cause
    (c) **T**
    (d) **F**
    (e) **T**

43. (a) **F** more females are affected F:M = 5:1
    (b) **F** topical steroids are of some value, and there is little evidence that systemic steroids change the course of the disease
    (c) **T**
    (d) **T** tuberculosis can provoke erythema nodosum
    (e) **F** it is an example of lymphocytic vasculitis

44. (a) **T**
    (b) **T**
    (c) **F**
    (d) **F**
    (e) **T** till recently cosmetic camouflage has been the treatment of choice; at present there is considerable interest in laser therapy, particularly for the adult-type lesions with central nodules which respond best

45. (a) T
(b) T
(c) T
(d) F
(e) T

46. (a) F hypohidrosis
(b) T
(c) T
(d) T
(e) F this is found in inflammatory bowel disease and rheumatoid arthritis

47. (a) T an inherited disorder of Zn-malabsorption; there is diarrhoea
(b) T associated with inflammatory bowel disease
(c) T familial adenomatosis polypi and mesodermal tumours
(d) T e.g. ulcerative colitis, tuberculosis, etc.
(e) T associated with coeliac disease

48. (a) T a histamine-releasing drug
(b) T e.g. benzoate
(c) T
(d) T
(e) T C_1-esterase inhibitor deficiency causes hereditary angio-oedema

49. (a) T
(b) F commoner
(c) T is associated with autoimmune diseases
(d) T
(e) F this is a feature of the hypopigmented macules of leprosy

50. (a) F
(b) T
(c) F
(d) T
(e) T

51. (a) T
(b) T this is the typical appearance of a dermatophyte infection after it has been aggravated by steroids
(c) T
(d) F these are thin white lines on the surface of lichen planus
(e) F in this disease there is an enzymatic defect in the repair–replication of DNA in the skin predisposing to keratoses and malignancies after solar exposure

52. (a) **F** koilonychia 'spoon-shaped nails' is a feature of iron deficiency anaemia
(b) **T** single transverse depression on the nails due to temporary interference with nail formation due to a serious illness such as myocardial infarction, pneumonia, etc.
(c) **F**
(d) **F** chloroquine therapy may produce a blue/black discoloration of nails
(e) **F** blue/black discoloration may be due to antimalarials, phenothiazines or subungual haematoma

53. All **T**

54. (a) **F** this is intra-epidermal
(b) **T**
(c) **T**
(d) **F** this is intra-epidermal
(e) **T**

55. (a) **T**
(b) **T**
(c) **F** only in few cases
(d) **F** usually on the trunk
(e) **F** adequate excision is the treatment of choice

56. (a) **F**
(b) **T**
(c) **F** fortunately it is rare
(d) **F** this is uncommon in the UK
(e) **F**

57. (a) **T**
(b) **F** this is a feature of tertiary syphilis
(c) **T**
(d) **T**
(e) **F** this is a feature of tertiary syphilis

58. (a) **F**
(b) **T**
(c) **T**
(d) **T**
(e) **T**

59. (a) **T**
 (b) **F** it is much less common
 (c) **F** prednisolone for widespread acute disease and potent topical steroids for less acute cases
 (d) **T**
 (e) **F** the disease commonly lasts for 18–24 months

60. (a) **F** females are commonly affected
 (b) **F** potent steroids should not be used on the face
 (c) **F** comedones are characteristic of acne
 (d) **T** hypertrophic tissue can be shaven from nose
 (e) **T**

61. (a) **F** least common in Japan
 (b) **T**
 (c) **F** these are typically involved
 (d) **T**
 (e) **F** chloroquine should be avoided as it aggravates the skin lesions

62. (a) **T**
 (b) **T**
 (c) **T**
 (d) **T**
 (e) **T** this syndrome is associated with iron-deficiency anaemia and koilonychia (usually females affected)

63. (a) **T**
 (b) **T**
 (c) **F**
 (d) **F**
 (e) **T**

64. (a) **T**
 (b) **F** UVR exacerbates the condition
 (c) **T**
 (d) **F** no effect
 (e) **T**

65. (a) **T** this is a form of bullous pemphigoid
 (b) **T**
 (c) **F** this is seen in rheumatic fever
 (d) **F**
 (e) **T**

66. (a) F *Trichophyton rubrum, T. interdigitale,* and *Epidermophyton floccosum* are most commonly implicated
    (b) F if nail-pitting is present, psoriasis is the likely diagnosis
    (c) T
    (d) T
    (e) T treatment needs to be prolonged, up to 9 months for finger-nails and up to 2 years for toe-nails

67. (a) F was described in 1874
    (b) F very occasionally the intraduct carcinoma is absent
    (c) T loss of the nipple is a good physical sign that helps to differentiate from eczema
    (d) T
    (e) F

68. (a) F this is due to *M. leprae*
    (b) T
    (c) T also called Bazin's disease
    (d) F this is an exaggeration of the ridge pattern of the palm seen in acanthosis nigricans
    (e) T

69. (a) F this is caused by *Erysipelothrix insidiosa*
    (b) T
    (c) T
    (d) F due to *Corynebacterium minutissimum*
    (e) F probably due to a virus

70. (a) T
    (b) T
    (c) T
    (d) F this is a neurological syndrome of failure of pupillary convergence reflex with failure of up gaze
    (e) T

71. (a) T
    (b) F
    (c) T
    (d) T
    (e) F

72. (a) F steroids should not be used
    (b) F this responds to imidazoles or Selsum shampoo
    (c) F this is aggravated by steroids (herpes simplex infection)
    (d) F this is aggravated by steroids
    (e) F

73. All **T**

74.
- (a) **T**
- (b) **T**
- (c) **T** the third component of the response is particularly exaggerated
- (d) **F**
- (e) **T**

75.
- (a) **F** this is the commonest cutaneous disease due to tuberculosis
- (b) **F** this is a benign adenoma of sweat glands
- (c) **T** this is the commonest cutaneous manifestation
- (d) **F** this is a skin infection due to a skin commensal
- (e) **F** this is a 'heat rash' due to blockage to sweat ducts by overhydrated keratin in hot climates

76.
- (a) **T**
- (b) **F** this is caused by a coxsackie virus
- (c) **F** this is genital warts caused by human papilloma virus
- (d) **T** this classically develops in atopics and resembles varicella
- (e) **F** this syndrome is caused by the varicella virus

77. All **T**

78.
- (a) **T**
- (b) **T**
- (c) **F** see 75 (e)
- (d) **F**
- (e) **F**

79. All **T**

80.
- (a) **F** 'café-au-lait' macules are characteristic
- (b) **F** hyperpigmented macules around the mouth with intestinal polyps
- (c) **T** *Malassezia furfur* produces azaleic acid which bleaches melanin
- (d) **T** this is a form of dermatitis seen in children
- (e) **T** there are hypopigmented anaesthetic macules in tuberculoid leprosy

81. (a) F hypopigmentation results from hypopituitarism
    (b) T due to raised ACTH and raised β-MSH (there is a loss of negative feedback exerted by cortisol) this is true in primary hypoadrenalism only
    (c) T
    (d) F there is generalized hypopigmentation due to a defect in phenylalanine-4-hydroxylase
    (e) F this is patchy hyperpigmentation (e.g. in the axillae) which usually indicates (in an adult) an underlying malignancy

82. (a) F it emits long-wave UVR
    (b) F
    (c) T
    (d) T
    (e) T

83. (a) F autosomal dominant
    (b) T
    (c) T
    (d) T
    (e) F

84. (a) F
    (b) F hypotonia is a feature
    (c) T
    (d) T
    (e) T

85. (a) F this is a feature of tertiary syphilis
    (b) T
    (c) T
    (d) F this is a feature of tertiary syphilis
    (e) T

86. (a) F this is exacerbated by sunlight
    (b) T
    (c) T
    (d) T
    (e) F the photosensitivity is precipitated by sunlight

87. (a) T
    (b) T
    (c) T
    (d) F
    (e) F

88. (a) **F**
(b) **T**
(c) **F** it is about 50%
(d) **F** less common
(e) **T** especially the oesophagus (abnormal peristalsis, reduced oesophageal sphincter pressure, strictures, etc.)

89. (a) **T**
(b) **T**
(c) **T**
(d) **T**
(e) **F** this causes thinning of the skin

90. (a) **T**
(b) **T** these mixtures contain iodides that may induce acne
(c) **T**
(d) **T** these are extensively used in the instillation industry
(e) **F**

91. (a) **F** only occasionally
(b) **T**
(c) **T** e.g. different penicillins, sulphonamides and hair dyes
(d) **F** gold-induced dermatosis may last for 7 months or longer
(e) **T**

92. (a) **T**
(b) **T**
(c) **F** this causes koilonychia
(d) **F** this may cause pitting, thickening, discoloration or onycholysis
(e) **T** in 10% of cases

93. (a) **F** this is usually due to venous hypertension
(b) **F** also known as nummular eczema
(c) **T**
(d) **F** there is a constitutional tendency but external factors such as irritants, infection, trauma ... contribute to it
(e) **F**

94. (a) **T**
(b) **T** after secondary involvement the liver becomes unable to degrade some of the tumour products such as 5HT which causes flushing
(c) **F**
(d) **T** this drug blocks Ca^{2+}-channels causing vasodilation
(e) **T**

55

95. (a) T
(b) F
(c) T
(d) T
(e) F

96. All **T**; all of these conditions can cause a sensory neuropathy

97. (a) **F** the hair loss is usually seen 2–4 months after a stressful event, e.g. shock, emotional upset, parturition, etc.
(b) **F** no treatment modality has been effective
(c) **F** these hairs may be seen in alopecia areata
(d) **T** these transverse lines are due to an arrest of the nail growth
(e) **T**

98. (a) **F** tryptophan is a precursor of nicotinamide
(b) **T** tryptophan is converted to other amines, e.g. 5HT rather than nicotinamide
(c) **F** very low protein diets may lead to pellagra
(d) **T** there is malabsorption of tryptophan (and other amino acids) and increased loss in urine
(e) **T** antagonizes Vit. B_6 which is required for the synthesis of nicotinamide

99. (a) **F**
(b) **T** this is carcinoma *in situ*
(c) **T**
(d) **T**
(e) **F** camouflaging creams and recently laser therapy have been successful

100. (a) **F**
(b) **T** the risk is increased by 15 times
(c) **F** this form is commoner in children and usually follows streptococcal tonsillitis
(d) **F** the extensor surfaces of elbows and knees are the commonest sites
(e) **F** no evidence

101. (a) **F** pemphigus vulgaris is commoner in Jews
(b) **T** e.g. prednisolone (50 mg per day), but other drugs can be used, e.g. azathioprine
(c) **T** mucosal membranes are rarely involved
(d) **F** sub-epidermal blisters (tense) are characteristic
(e) **F** the blisters are usually on the legs

102.
(a) **F** *B. anthracis* causes anthrax
(b) **T**
(c) **T** it is actually a tumour of proliferating dermal vessels (young capillaries) and bleeding after trauma can be troublesome
(d) **F**
(e) **F** cautery and curettage; it is important to send the specimen for histology to exclude a melanoma (amelanotic)

103. All **T**

104.
(a) **F** commoner in females
(b) **F** it should be differentiated from contact dermatitis before reassuring the patient
(c) **T**
(d) **T**
(e) **F** topical steroids (under polythene occlusion) are effective; sedatives may help

105.
(a) **F**
(b) **T** it is the commonest cutaneous disease due to *Mycobacterium tuberculosis*
(c) **F**
(d) **T**
(e) **T**

106.
(a) **F** Buruli ulcer is caused by *Mycobacterium ulcerans*
(b) **F** swimming pool granuloma (or fish tank granuloma) is caused by *M. marinum*
(c) **F** creeping eruption due to larvae of *Ancylostoma braziliense* and *Strongyloides stercoralis* mainly
(d) **F** epidermolysis bullosa is a congenital skin disease characterized by blisters; staphylococci can cause toxic epidermolysis in children
(e) **T**

107.
(a) **T** this accounts for 5% of cases
(b) **F**
(c) **T**
(d) **F**
(e) **F** erythema induratum is associated with tuberculosis especially in individuals with a strong delayed hypersensitivity reaction; erythema nodosum is the commonest cutaneous manifestation of sarcoidosis

108. (a) T
(b) T
(c) F this is oculocerebrorenal dystrophy with generalized amino aciduria
(d) T
(e) T

109. (a) F
(b) T
(c) T
(d) F diagnosis is usually made on clinical grounds
(e) T

110. (a) T (the scalp is often affected. The changes may simulate seborrhoeic dermatitis)
(b) T
(c) F
(d) F
(e) F

111. (a) T
(b) T
(c) T
(d) T
(e) F

112. (a) T
(b) T
(c) F this provokes itching; cotton underwear is recommended
(d) F salicylic acid is used in warts and skin hyperkeratosis (keratolytic agent)
(e) F this should never be tried

113. (a) F
(b) T
(c) T
(d) F
(e) F congenital erythroporphyria is autosomal recessive and erythropoietic protoporphyria is autosomal dominant

114. (a) T
(b) F hair becomes thin and may change colour to blond
(c) T
(d) T
(e) T

115. (a) T
(b) T
(c) T
(d) F
(e) F

116. (a) F
(b) T
(c) T
(d) F
(e) F

117. (a) T
(b) T
(c) F
(d) T
(e) T

118. (a) T to improve and maintain the functions of the hands and fingers
(b) T
(c) F
(d) F
(e) T

119. (a) F CPK levels are elevated due to muscle damage
(b) T
(c) T due to proximal muscle involvement
(d) F this is seen in pemphigus where new blisters form on applying pressure/rubbing on clinically normal skin
(e) T

120. All T

121. (a) T constipation is also occasionally seen
(b) F there is malabsorption of Zn^{2+} leading to low serum levels
(c) T
(d) F P. gangrenosum is associated with inflammatory bowel disease
(e) F

122. (a) T
(b) T
(c) F
(d) T
(e) T

123. (a) T
 (b) T
 (c) F commoner in black subjects
 (d) F the epidermis is normal
 (e) F

124. (a) F
 (b) T
 (c) T
 (d) T
 (e) F

125. (a) F
 (b) T
 (c) T
 (d) T
 (e) T

126. (a) T
 (b) T 'chemical cautery'
 (c) T
 (d) F see 117
 (e) F

127. (a) F (rare)
 (b) T
 (c) T
 (d) F (rare)
 (e) T 'eczema of hand and foot'

128. (a) T secondary infection is very common and there may be occipital lymphadenopathy
 (b) T
 (c) F
 (d) T
 (e) T

129. (a) T
 (b) F weak
 (c) F weak
 (d) F
 (e) T

130. (a) F
 (b) F
 (c) T
 (d) T
 (e) F

131. (a) **T**
(b) **F** this is caused by the yeast *Malassezia furfur*
(c) **F** griseofulvin is not effective against bacteria
(d) **F** this is the pork tapeworm; it causes human cysticercosis
(e) **F** griseofulvin is not effective against yeasts

132. (a) **F**
(b) **F**
(c) **F**
(d) **F**
(e) **T**

133. (a) **F** 'perniosis' is a feature of sarcoidosis
(b) **T**
(c) **F** results in impotence in a high proportion of cases
(d) **T**
(e) **T**

134. (a) **F** middle aged/elderly are usually affected
(b) **F**
(c) **T**
(d) **T** potent topical steroids, intralesional triamcinolone or impregnated steroid tapes are effective
(e) **F**

135. (a) **T**
(b) **T**
(c) **F** Koplik's spots are characteristic of measles
(d) **F** the vesicles are of different age
(e) **F**

136. (a) **F** the whites are usually spared
(b) **T** even in AIDS-related patients
(c) **F** is usually found in every organ except the brain in affected AIDS-patients; however, recently it has been reported in the brain
(d) **T** angiomas and glomus tumours also enter the differential diagnosis
(e) **T**

137. All **T**

138. (a) **F**
(b) **T**
(c) **T** e.g. Down's syndrome
(d) **F**
(e) **T**

139. (a) T
(b) T
(c) F
(d) T
(e) F

140. (a) F
(b) F
(c) F
(d) T
(e) F

141. All T

142. (a) T
(b) F *Haemophilus ducreyi* is sensitive to tetracycline and sulphonamides
(c) F
(d) F
(e) F

143. (a) T
(b) T
(c) T
(d) T
(e) T e.g. melanoma, squamous cell carcinoma, etc.

144. All T

145. All T

146. (a) T
(b) F
(c) T
(d) F
(e) T

147. (a) T
(b) T
(c) T
(d) T
(e) F

148. (a) T
     (b) F
     (c) F they are commonly found in normal people, but they increase in number in liver disease
     (d) F they are dilated capillaries
     (e) T

149. (a) T
     (b) F
     (c) F
     (d) F
     (e) T

150. (a) T
     (b) T
     (c) T
     (d) F this is usually seen on the lower limbs as painful erythematous nodules
     (e) F this is usually seen on the face of patients with tuberous sclerosis

151. (a) F caused by *Leishmania mexicam*, found in America
     (b) F caused by *L. amazonensis* (America)
     (c) T caused by *L. tropica minor* (oriental sore)
     (d) F caused by *L. braziliensis* (America)
     (e) F caused by *L. peruviana* (Andes)

152. (a) T
     (b) T
     (c) F smallpox vaccine is contra-indicated
     (d) F commoner in cow's milk feeding
     (e) F

153. (a) F lower incidence is associated with early circumcision (at birth of Jews)
     (b) F elderly subjects
     (c) T
     (d) T
     (e) F there is groin lymphadenopathy in 60% of cases some of which is inflammatory in nature

154. (a) T in a study in Finland 1 in 7 patients with hepatoma had porphyria
     (b) F the abnormal enzyme protoporphyrinogen oxidase
     (c) F a bullous eruption appears on sun-exposure
     (d) F is an acute hepatic porphyria
     (e) F the onset is usually in adolescence

155. (a) F
 (b) F males are more frequently affected (M:F = 3:1)
 (c) T this antigen is occasionally found in the immune complex, but in most cases the antigen is unknown
 (d) F this syndrome refers to the association of scleroderma, calcinosis and widespread telengiectasia
 (e) T due to mononeuritis multiplex

156. All T

157. (a) F this is cortical blindness syndrome due to bilateral occipital damage
 (b) T
 (c) T
 (d) F
 (e) T

158. (a) F the serum iron and transferrin saturation are usually raised
 (b) T
 (c) F
 (d) T
 (e) T alcohol is the commonest precipitating agent

159. (a) F
 (b) T
 (c) F
 (d) F
 (e) T

160. (a) T
 (b) T
 (c) F this causes generalized hypopigmentation
 (d) F
 (e) F this is a precursor of melanoma; it is flat freckle-like lesions due to presence of melanocytes at epidermo-dermal junction

161. (a) F mainly 10–40 years of age
 (b) F
 (c) T usually 60 years
 (d) F in young adults and children
 (e) T

162. (a) F the patients are usually children, adolescents or young adults
     (b) T usually type I (accounts for about 30% of cases)
     (c) T an ophthalmological opinion should be sought early to prevent serious eye complications
     (d) T
     (e) F the lesions (concentric erythematous papules) are usually seen on the back of the hands, forearms, feet and toes

163. (a) F
     (b) T
     (c) T
     (d) F
     (e) T

164. (a) T
     (b) F
     (c) T
     (d) T
     (e) F squamous cell carcinoma

165. (a) F is usually caused by *Streptococcus pyogenes*
     (b) T
     (c) F systemic antibiotics are required to avoid septicaemia
     (d) F
     (e) T

166. (a) T
     (b) T
     (c) F
     (d) T
     (e) T

167. (a) T
     (b) T
     (c) F it can be treated by intralesional triamcinolone
     (d) F in one study about 70% of cases were below the age of 30 years
     (e) T

168. (a) F they are due to human papilloma viruses (HPV)
     (b) T
     (c) F
     (d) F
     (e) T

169. (a) T
(b) F it is usually due to a *single* exposure to a *strong* irritant, while allergic contact eczema is due to exposure to a mild irritant causing allergy
(c) F history-taking is most important
(d) T
(e) T due to use of irritants such as detergents

170. (a) F
(b) T
(c) T
(d) F surgery is the treatment of choice
(e) F

171. (a) F these are an important feature of neurofibromatosis
(b) F this is seen in pityriasis rosea
(c) T this is subcutaneous bruising seen through the skin around the umbilicus
(d) T this is subcutaneous bruising seen at the flanks
(e) T

172. (a) T
(b) T
(c) F this is retinocerebellar angiomatosis which is inherited in a dominant fashion
(d) T
(e) T

173. All F

174. (a) F this is a feature of tertiary syphilis
(b) F this is a feature of tertiary syphilis (neurosyphilis)
(c) F
(d) T
(e) T

175. (a) F in one study atopy was present in 18% of children with alopecia areata; if atopy is present the prognosis is worse
(b) T
(c) F usually, there are no subjective symptoms and the localized hair loss is first noticed by a relative or hairdresser
(d) T other autoimmune diseases may be present
(e) F alopecia totalis develops in about 8% of cases

176. (a) **F** it is aggravated by sunlight
(b) **T**
(c) **F**
(d) **T**
(e) **T**

177. (a) **T**
(b) **T**
(c) **T**
(d) **F** this refers to hair loss secondary to hair being broken from self-induced trauma
(e) **T**

178. (a) **T**
(b) **F** skin is involved in 10% of cases
(c) **T** anterior uveitis may be found in about 25% of cases
(d) **F** hypercalcaemia in 10% of cases
(e) **F** fatality rate in American blacks is about 8% compared with 4% in UK subjects

179. (a) **F** it is a rare photodermatosis of unknown aetiology; Hutchinson's teeth are a feature of late congenital syphilis
(b) **F** the rash begins as grouped papules on sun-exposed areas; non-exposed areas may be involved
(c) **T**
(d) **T**
(e) **T**

180. (a) **F**
(b) **T**
(c) **F**
(d) **F** these are mucous membrane manifestations of secondary syphilis (oropharynx and genitals)
(e) **T**

181. All **T**

182. (a) **F** this is a cytotoxic drug
(b) **F** this is a potent steroid that should not be used on the face
(c) **T** 1% in a cream base
(d) **T**
(e) **F** this is antifungal

183. All **T**

184.   (a) **F** this has no cutaneous manifestations
     (b) **T**
     (c) **T**
     (d) **T**
     (e) **F** this is a syndrome of generalized hyperpigmentation associated with an enlarging tumour after bilateral adrenalectomy

185.   (a) **F** 15% only
     (b) **F** 10% only
     (c) **F** 5% only
     (d) **T** over 85% of cases
     (e) **F** 10% only

186.   (a) **T**
     (b) **F**
     (c) **F**
     (d) **F** this is a treatment modality for alopecia
     (e) **T**

187.   (a) **F** it is extremely rare before this age
     (b) **T**
     (c) **T**
     (d) **F** surgery is indicated if conservative measures fail
     (e) **F** this is radical nail-bed ablation

188.   All **T**

189.   (a) **F**
     (b) **F**
     (c) **T**
     (d) **F**
     (e) **T**

190.   (a) **F** lepromin test is strongly positive
     (b) **F** due to *Mycobacterium leprae*
     (c) **F** very few acid-fast bacilli
     (d) **T** facial lesions are not usually anaesthetic
     (e) **F** there is loss of hair and sweating at the site of the lesion

191.   (a) **T**
     (b) **F** hyperkeratosis
     (c) **F** the epidermal transit time is decreased
     (d) **T**
     (e) **T** occasionally neutrophils invade the epidermis due to chemotaxis and form micro-abscesses (pustular)

192. (a) T
    (b) T e.g. carcinoid syndrome
    (c) T e.g. leukaemia
    (d) F
    (e) F

193. (a) F this is a benign adenoma of eccrine sweat glands
    (b) F
    (c) T
    (d) T
    (e) T

194. (a) F crust is dried exudate
    (b) F ecchymosis is a large bruise
    (c) F it is a flat circumscribed area of discoloration
    (d) T
    (e) T

195. (a) F this is a characteristic feature of DLE
    (b) T refers to retention of nuclei by immature corneocytes
    (c) F these vessels usually dilate in eczema
    (d) T
    (e) T

196. (a) F
    (b) T
    (c) T
    (d) F
    (e) F

197. (a) F it is teratogenic
    (b) T
    (c) T
    (d) F
    (e) F

198. (a) F acquired ichthyosis may complicate lymphoma
    (b) T this is an unusual manifestation (on the lower limbs)
    (c) T
    (d) T 'diabetic dermopathy'
    (e) T

199. (a) F this is a benign overgrowth of sebaceous tissue
    (b) T
    (c) T the creamy discharge dries up in the centre forming a sebaceous horn
    (d) T
    (e) T

200. (a) **F** autosomal dominant mode
(b) **F** due to deficiency of C_1-esterase inhibitor
(c) **T**
(d) **T**
(e) **T**

201. (a) **T** not always
(b) **T** not always
(c) **F** if anything it tends to improve (physiological hypercortisonism)
(d) **T** it occurs more frequently and spreads more widely
(e) **F** if anything it tends to improve

202. (a) **F** is made worse with steroids
(b) **F**
(c) **F** is made worse with steroids
(d) **F** stretch marks are irreversible and can be caused by steroids
(e) **F** infections are aggravated by steroids

203. (a) **F** this is the infantile analogue of adult dandruff
(b) **F** this is the photosensitivity of pallagra
(c) **T**
(d) **T**
(e) **F** these are transverse depressions on the nails (myocardial infarction, pneumonia, etc.)

204. (a) **F** this causes blue/black nails
(b) **T** the nails may also be thickened
(c) **T**
(d) **F** this causes transverse white bands in nails (white nails)
(e) **F** these drugs cause blue/black discoloration of nails

205. (a) **F** there is senile sebaceous hypertrophy
(b) **T** the epidermal cells become smaller, the corneocytes become larger and the sweating decreases (partially accounting for this)
(c) **T** multifactorial
(d) **T**
(e) **F** sweating paradoxically decreases

206. (a) **F** there is no evidence of systemic involvement
(b) **F**
(c) **F** lichen amyloidosis is another cutaneous (only) form
(d) **T**
(e) **T**

207. (a) T (swimming)
(b) F this is a syndrome of vitiligo, alopecia areata and uveitis
(c) F this is generalized pustular psoriasis
(d) T yachting, horse-riding and swimming (in the sea)
(e) T sporting in hot humid weather

208. (a) T
(b) T
(c) T
(d) T
(e) F this is a condition of the elderly and may be confused with ankylosing spondylitis

209. (a) T
(b) T
(c) T
(d) F this is localized sclerosis of the skin
(e) F this is a spinal muscular atrophy seen in childhood

210. (a) F
(b) F it is a mass of young capillaries
(c) T
(d) T especially if the melanoma is amelanocytic and rapidly growing
(e) T

211. (a) F caused by a pox virus
(b) T this occurs if the lesion is incized and antigen is released
(c) F settle in about 7 weeks
(d) F milker's nodes are caused by another pox virus which is very similar (morphologically) to that causing orf
(e) T

212. (a) T this is spastic diplegia, mental retardation and ichthyotic skin
(b) T the pigmented epidermal naevi are associated with epilepsy/mental retardation in this syndrome
(c) F these are red spots (keratoangiomas), seen on the trunk and limbs with increasing frequency throughout middle age
(d) T associated with epilepsy and severe mental retardation
(e) T this is port-wine naevus on the face and a leptomeningeal angioma; it is associated with epilepsy

213.
(a) **T** especially if pH is low
(b) **F** these are tiny papules on the cheeks and the nose and are due to blocked sebaceous ducts
(c) **T** neck, face, and scalp (cradle cap) are also affected; it usually begins before the age of 3 months and is gone by 9 months
(d) **T** washing powders and ammonia are examples
(e) **F** this refers to red facies seen in some diabetics; it is thought to be due to microangiopathy

214.
(a) **F** varicose ulceration is due to venous hypertension
(b) **T**
(c) **T**
(d) **T**
(e) **T**

215.
(a) **T**
(b) **T**
(c) **T** there is amino aciduria and pellagra (defective absorption of tryptophan from the gastrointestinal tract and the renal tubule)
(d) **T** renal tumours are found in about 40% of cases (usually angiomyolipoma)
(e) **T**

216.
(a) **T**
(b) **T**
(c) **F** this reaction is positive in tuberculoid leprosy
(d) **T**
(e) **T** it is also associated with giantism and hyperthyroidism

217.
(a) **T** this is a limited form of polyarthritis nodosa which produces asthma; the lungs, peripheral nerves, the skin (tender subcutaneous nodules, purpura, petechiae and ulcers) and kidneys may be affected
(b) **T** sulphonamide can produce asthma and cause various skin reactions, e.g. allergic vasculitis, erythema nodosum, erythema multiforme, etc.
(c) **T** acanthosis nigricans, herpes zoster, dermatomyositus and clubbing are recognized cutaneous manifestations of this tumour
(d) **T** tuberous sclerosis is a recognized cause of a diffuse honeycomb lung
(e) **T**

218.
(a) **F** commoner in children
(b) **F** aspirin is a histamine-releasing drug that may precipitate attacks of flushing and irritation of the skin
(c) **T** the lesions are sparse on the limbs
(d) **T** there is an increase in the number of mast cells in the skin
(e) **F** the adult is less likely to lose the disease; it usually occurs in children and fades in late childhood

219.
(a) **F** steroids have been shown to be disadvantageous in children
(b) **T** painful lesions with systemic symptoms require high dose steroids (80–100 mg)
(c) **T**
(d) **F** this is self-limiting; penicillin maybe given for a week
(e) **F** in fact systemic steroids may cause acne

220.
(a) **F** aortic regurgitation occurs due to a dilated aortic ring; the mitral valve may be similarly affected
(b) **T** this is due to joint laxity; if the thumb is abducted across the palm its tip is seen to cross the ulnar border of the palm
(c) **T** this is the only common dermatological feature
(d) **F** this is a dilated pupil (myotonic) seen in young females due to denervation of the ciliary body; it usually has no pathological significance
(e) **T**